AMAZING AT 50: 10-DAY FLAT TUMMY CHALLENGE

QUICK & EASY WORKOUTS PLUS 14-DAY MEAL PLAN

I. NGEOW

978-1-913584-02-3

Written and illustrated by I. Ngeow

First published in Great Britain in 2020 by Leopard Print

CONTENTS

INTRODUCTION

CONGRATULATIONS ON MAKING THE first step. You're taking responsibility for your own health and fitness. Beginning is 80% of your goal. Completing it is the other 20%. Somewhere in between is where you can see your goal.

Your equipment list consists of this book, your own bodyweight, your mind.

I am an ordinary suburban working mom. Inside this book are no gimmicks, drugs, gadgets, Photoshop or filters. The photos you see in this book are snapshots and have not been retouched. I am all real and proud to be the age and the woman that I am. It took me 50 years to be this awesome. I don't see the purpose of photographic tricks.

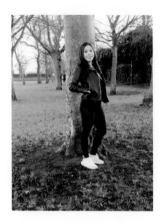

ESTABLISH YOUR AIMS AND OBJECTIVES

Most people give up on fitness and nutrition too quickly. Why? Because they never commit to one thing at a time. They want to do it all and they want it all, now. They want results today. There is no such thing.

We want to avoid such shocks to your body. One small step, giant leap etc. Always work methodically and put in your best effort each time. You will see guaranteed results.

HOW DO YOU KNOW IF YOU ARE FIT AND HEALTHY?

By the size of your waist. Forget everything else. The old common sense cliches are true: "keeping an eye on the waistline", "watching the middle-age spread," "losing an inch" etc.

"Keeping your waist circumference to less than half your height can help increase life expectancy for every person in the world," said Dr Margaret Ashwell[1], former science director of the British Nutrition Foundation. "The ratio was also better than just taking a waist measurement, as it took into account differing height between individuals and ethnic groups."

The team, who analyzed the health of some 300,000 people, found this ratio was a better predictor of high blood pressure, diabetes and cardiovascular events like heart attacks and strokes than body mass index.

Traditionally the Body Mass Index (BMI) has been used as an indicator of life expectancy and obesity. But BMI does not take into account the distribution of abdominal fat, around the heart, liver and kidneys, which has been found to be worse than that on the bottom and hips, in terms of heart disease and diabetes. BMI is calculated by taking one's mass in kilograms and dividing it by the square of one's height in metres.

Dr Ashwell said that waist-to-height ratio should be considered as a screening tool. Grab your tape measure now and do this simple test. For example:

If you are 6' (72") tall man, your waist measurement should be less than 36".

If you are a 5' 6" (66") tall woman your waist measurement should be less than 33".

The second indicator of your fitness and health is wearing off-the-shelf clothes. For your height and clothes size, are your clothes pinching you at the waist?

Watch the inches and the pounds will take care of themselves.

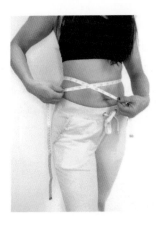

---

1. Adams, Stephen, Medical Correspondent, "Forget BMI, Just Measure Your Waist and Height", *The Daily Telegraph*, 12 May 2012

FREQUENTLY ASKED QUESTIONS

1. WILL I LOSE FAT AND SLIM DOWN?

You WILL. HIIT (see below) is how you burn fat. But the amount will depend on your age, previous training, genetics, how you're sleeping, what you're eating and how hard you exercise. The aim is to be healthier and leaner, and therefore any progress will be an improvement.

2. WHAT IS HIIT?

High Intensity Interval Training is short bursts of intense exercise (also called cardio) followed by short rest periods. Repeat this pattern and that's it. HIIT burns calories for up to 18 hours afterwards even when you are not exercising such as when you are sleeping! Isn't that the best news? During your recovery, your body is working hard to repay the oxygen debt in your systems and restore itself to a resting stage. Your metabolic rate rises during the rest period so your body is burning more fat or more calories. During the intense part, work yourself hard as passible, so hard that you cannot speak. The harder you work the greater the oxygen debt therefore the more fat you will burn during the rest period.

3. ARE THESE EXERCISES FOR EVERYBODY?

Absolutely. Check first with your doctor if you have any health issues. The exercises are simple to follow. The first two sessions will be hard if you have never exercised before or have had a prolonged break. If it's too easy, work harder and if it's too hard, take a break or work less hard, but come back again and give it your best shot.

4. HOW DO I STAY MOTIVATED?

You can train with a friend or you can reward yourself after each session by giving yourself something pleasant (not food). If you do not want to do something, pay yourself. Put money in a jar and label the jar "shoe fund" or "holiday fund", for example. I believe in rewards. We reward children for good behaviour and it is how we train our minds and not just our bodies. Our body will start to obey. And in fact, after the first two weeks, guess what? You will start to see results and there is no greater motivation than results. Measure and weigh yourself before you start the plan. Also take photos of your front and side views in a swimsuit, underwear or bikini. Repeat in a month. Once you see yourself transformed, don't worry, you will be motivated.

5. WHAT SHOULD I DO BEFORE I START?

Book the time in, just as though you have meetings that you cannot miss. See the exercise journal section at the back of this book and fill the table in. Yes, you have very important meetings and it's with yourself. You are your own project. See it as beauty appointments or hospital treatments. Take it seriously. Don't leave it to chance or the table blank. You commit to it by writing it down. Keep track and count all your rounds. Each one takes you a step closer to being fit and lean.

6. DO I HAVE TO EAT WHAT'S ON THE MEAL PLAN?

You should but you don't have to stick to it religiously. It is an Asian-style portion control guide, and it's more like "trying on for size" only. Once you start eating less and cutting out the junk (sugar, high fat, high salt processed food, takeouts, instant supermarket meals, which means anything that comes in batter, a box or a bag), you won't feel like eating unhealthy food again. The meal plan is to only to help you avoid processed and/or junk food. With a regime or routine, it's easier not to be led astray or randomly eat because you have a plan that you will always be able to refer to. And then when you *do* go to restaurants or buy takeouts, you are much more aware that it is a total treat in itself and in fact you are probably a much better cook than the chef!

7. DO YOU HAVE ANY TIPS FOR EATING LESS?

Do not finish your children's or spouse's meals (which I have been known to do, since I am Asian). Save those for another mini meal, if you, like me, don't throw away food.

You'll also save money because you can stretch unfinished meals to another meal. No one ever told you that but it's absolutely common sense and true. Save money and slim down! It was how our forefathers survived from day to day in hard times, by splitting meals, eating half and saving the other half.

Drink water before eating. It will help you eat less because maybe you are actually thirsty. Always think before you put something in your mouth. Are you actually hungry or are you sad, bored, thirsty or all three? Build a relationship with food based on good habits.

Don't associate food with emotional needs. Think of the food you are eating rather than eating the food you are thinking of. You will NOT be hungry, because when you are hungry you WILL eat well.

It is eating badly that makes you hungry. Hence the vicious circle. The great news is that exercise curbs your appetite. Pair that with healthy eating and you have a winning combination.

8. WHAT IF I'M TOO BUSY TO EXERCISE?

I am a busy working mom myself. That is why this plan has been designed. This is a customized workout for the time-poor.

"Fit in fitness to be fit." - Ivy Ngeow

---

9. WHAT IF I DON'T LIKE EXERCISE?

You only don't like it because a) you ate the wrong things, b) you saw no difference and c) you gave up too soon. If you get all three right, it's a win-win. You will never dislike it again. In fact, you will love it so much you won't want to stop and you'll wonder why you didn't like it. Really.

THE WORKOUT PLAN

THE PLAN IS BASED on 5 days a week of exercise for 2 weeks. Allocate the time by writing it in your exercise journal, calendar or timetable.

This plan is a high intensity interval training (HIIT) program which will both burn fat and add definition. Before you begin make sure you have

- an exercise mat
- T-shirt and shorts or leggings and a good sports bra
- a bottle of water
- an app timer on a phone or an old-fashioned timer. a towel (optional)

If you have not exercised before, then this is a great way to start as the workouts are designed to help you push yourself.

I am half-a-century year old working mom, a qualified writer, architect, makeup artist and musician. I am not a doctor, personal trainer or dietician. But I know what works on me, and it's being consistent with the program and the nutrition.

You need very little space. You can do these exercises in your bedroom at home, a hotel room, a park, a poolside, anywhere. Just take this book with you.

If you're ready, let's begin.

WEEK ONE

DAY 1

- 10 straight leg raises
- 10 sit-ups
- 10 crunches
- 20 heel touches (10 per side)
- 16 high knee running (8 per side)
- 10 squats
- 10 burpees
- 20 second plank

DAY 2

- 20 jumping jacks
- 20 alternating lunges (10 per side)
- 5 push ups
- 20 butt kicks (10 per side)
- 12 sit ups

- 12 crunches
- 12 leg raises
- 16 scissor/flutter kicks (8 per side)

DAY 3

- 30 ab bikes (15 per side)
- 15 burpees
- 25 second plank
- 15 sit-ups
- 24 heel touches (10 per side)
- 6 push ups
- 20 high knee running
- 15 leg raises

DAY 4

- 10 sitting twists or Russian Twists (5 per side)[1]
- 7 push ups
- 20 mountain climbers (10 per side)
- 30 second plank
- 15 tricep dips
- 15 squats
- 15 crunches
- 20 leg raises

DAY 5

- 40 second plank
- 20 crunches
- 30 scissor/flutter kicks
- 14 Russian Twists (7 per side)

- 20 reverse lunges (10 per side)
- 28 high knee running (14 per side)
- 30 ab bikes (15 per side)

DAY 6 and DAY 7: REST

---

1. Hot tip: While doing Russian Twist, holding something a bit heavy, eg a laptop, 2 bottles or water, 2 bags of flour or 2 little dumbbells/hand weights, and it can be whatever that gives a little resistance but not too heavy or too light.

WEEK TWO

DAY 8

- Side plank (10 sec per side)
- 20 sit-ups
- Reverse lunges (10 per leg)
- 30 heel touches (15 per side)
- 15 straight leg raises
- 15 burpees
- 20 high knee running (10 per side)
- 20 crunches

DAY 9

- 20 jumping jacks
- 20 alternating front lunges (10 per side)
- 10 push ups
- 20 butt kicks (10 per side)
- 20 sit ups

- 20 crunches
- 15 leg raises
- 20 scissor/flutter kicks (10 per side)

DAY 10

- 40 mountain climbers
- Side plank (15 sec per side)
- 20 sit ups
- 20 straight leg raises with hip raise
- 20 reverse lunges (10 per side)
- 30 high knee running (10 per side)
- 20 crunches
- 20 jumping jacks

DAY 11

- 40 high knee running (20 per side)
- 30 ab bikes
- 40 scissor/flutter kicks (20 per side)
- 5 push ups
- 30 sec plank
- 25 squats
- 20 straight leg raises with hip raise
- 10 Russian Twists

DAY 12

- 40 second plank
- 20 crunches
- 40 scissor/flutter kicks
- 20 straight leg raises with hip raise

- 20 reverse lunges (10 per side)
- 30 high knee running (15 per side)
- 30 ab bikes (15 per side)

DAY 13 and DAY 14: REST

DAY 15

CONGRATULATIONS, you made it! Treat yourself and have another day off or begin straightaway on Awesome at 50: Body Reboot in 6 weeks.

NUTRITION GUIDE

DREAM (DON'T REPEATEDLY EAT AS MUCH) is an acronym I invented. DREAM is the natural, simple and sensible way to eat your way to great health, and the way it was always meant to be.

You can eat whatever you want within reason, and you will still stay slim. "Within reason" means the amount that you eat should be proportional to you. We were born to feed ourselves with our own hands. Therefore, our hand size is all that is required to measure what we put in our mouths.

The guideline works like this:

- your protein in each meal should be fist-sized,
- carbs palm-sized, and
- vegetables or salad the size of two fists.

A cup size is roughly a fist. However, we all have different sized fists! So please adjust accordingly to your own anatomy.

5 quick rules:

- *cut out the excess sugar and salt from your diet. You will see an IMMEDIATE body change.*
- *portion your meals out (have your big three meals of the day but in-between eat a healthy snack. Almonds are a healthy snack but 10 handful of almonds do more harm than good,*
- *cut out the junk food as snacks,*
- *find a healthy snack you can enjoy that gets rid of the junk food craving and remember to*
- *keep up with your workouts.*

You do not have to follow the meal plan exactly, as mentioned in the FAQs. The idea is to replace it with a similar item in both portion and nutrition. Don't worry, you can cheat! Your body is clever and so are you. You can get back on track the next day. Do not cheat more than once a week otherwise you are defeating the purpose of the intensive workout.

14-DAY MEAL PLAN

DAY 1

Breakfast

4 boiled eggs

1 large grapefruit

Protein shake

Snack

25 almonds

Lunch

Shrimp and quinoa lettuce wraps

1 cup of salad with 2 tbsp oil/vinegar dressing

Protein bar

1 apple

Snack

1 piece of string cheese[1]

Dinner

Chicken curry w/ 1 cup of brown rice

Half cup of vegetables

DAY 2

Breakfast
2 tbsp of peanut butter with 1 piece of toast
1 banana
Protein bar
Snack
2 small boxes of raisins
Lunch
Leftover chicken curry
1 cup salad
wholewheat pitta or naan bread
Snack
0% fat Greek yogurt
Shake
Dinner
Char siew grilled pork chops
1 cup of brown rice
1 cup of cucumber

DAY 3

Breakfast
4 scrambled eggs with ham or cheese
1 large grapefruit
Snack
25 almonds
Lunch
Udon noodles with leftover grilled pork chops

1 cup spinach

1 apple

Snack

2 pieces of string cheese

Dinner

Eggplant and okra (or sugar snap peas) sambal

1 cup of salad with walnut oil dressing

Brown basmati pilau rice

DAY 4

Breakfast

3 high protein low carb waffles w/ ¼ dsp syrup

0% fat Greek yogurt

Snack

1 cup snap peas

4 Tbsp of hummus

Lunch

Leftover eggplant and okra sambal curry

Half cup sugar snap peas

1 wholewheat naan bread or pitta bread

1 apple

Snack

1 banana

1 piece of string cheese

Shake

Dinner

2 cups of shrimp, Chinese cabbage and carrots

1 cup of quinoa

2 cups of spinach

DAY 5

Breakfast

2 tbsp of peanut butter in brown toasted sandwich

0% fat Greek yogurt

1 large grapefruit

Snack

1 pear

Lunch

Leftover shrimp, cabbage and carrots

1 cup of salad

25 almonds

Protein shake

Snack

30 baby carrots

1 boiled egg

Dinner

1 cup fish curry

1 cup of spinach

1 cup of brown rice

2 cups of green beans

DAY 6

Breakfast

4 egg-loaded vegetable omelet

1 banana

Snack

3 mozzarella pearls

Shake

Lunch

Fish curry leftovers with salad

Protein Bar

1 apple

Snack

10 cherry tomatoes

2 tbsp of hummus

Dinner

Eat out

Dessert

Sugar-free ice cream

DAY 7

Breakfast

Oatmeal

1 banana

Snack

15 baby carrots

2 Tbsp of hummus

Lunch

Eat out

Snack

0% fat Greek yogurt

Protein shake

Dinner

2 cups wholewheat penne with chopped chicken in pesto 2 cups of spinach

DAY 8

Breakfast
3 scrambled eggs
1 large grapefruit
Snack
25 almonds
Lunch
Turkey wholewheat wrap
1 apple
Snack
4 mozzarella pearls
Dinner
Spicy chicken and wholewheat pasta
Side salad and 2 tbsp olive oil/vinegar dressing

DAY 9

Breakfast
2 tbsp of peanut butter with 1 piece of toast
1 banana
Snack
2 small boxes of raisins
Lunch
Leftovers
Snack
0% fat Greek yogurt
Dinner
Miso salmon
2 cups of broccoli

DAY 10

Breakfast
Lean eggs and ham

1 large grapefruit

Snack
25 almonds

Lunch
Black bean and cheese burrito

1 apple

Snack
1 piece of string cheese

Dinner
Veggie Burger and bun

Salad with 4 Tbsp olive oil/vinegar dressing

1 serving of sweet potato fries

DAY 11

Breakfast
Berry wholewheat wafflewich

0% fat Greek yogurt

Snack
15 snap peas

2 Tbsp of hummus

Lunch
Sandwich

1 apple

Snack
1 banana

1 piece of string cheese

Dinner

Steamed Snapper with Pesto
1 cup of brown rice
2 cups of broccoli

DAY 12

Breakfast
0% fat Greek yogurt
1 large grapefruit
Snack
Granola bar
Lunch
Salad
25 almonds
Snack
20-30 baby carrots
4 Tbsp of hummus
Dinner
Chicken Spinach Parm
1 cup of brown rice
2 cups of snow peas

DAY 13

Breakfast
Loaded Vegetable Omelet
1 banana
Snack
1 piece of string cheese
Lunch
Turkey Wholewheat Wrap
1 apple

Snack

10 cherry tomatoes

2 Tbsp of hummus

Dinner

Quick Lemon Chicken with Rice

2 cups of broccoli

Snack

Sugar-Free ice-cream

DAY 14

Breakfast

Loaded Vegetable Omelet

1 banana

Snack

15 baby carrots

2 Tbsp of hummus

Lunch

Eat Out

Snack

0% fat Greek yogurt

Dinner

Penne with Chicken Marengo

2 cups of broccoli

---

1. String cheese is string mozzarella. Throughout the plan, you can substitute it with mozzarella pearls, vegan mozzarella or tofu. Do not mistake it for Cheestrings which is a kids' cheese snack.

EXERCISE JOURNAL

Jot down the week, day and date. Check each day off as = "done" in the last column.

#success !

For example:

Done

WEEK ONE
Monday 03/16
Tuesday 03/17
Wednesday
Thursday
Friday
WEEK TWO
Monday
Tuesday
Wednesday
Thursday
Friday

ILLUSTRATIONS

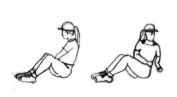

Sitting twists.

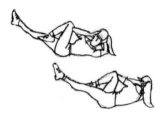

Ab bikes.

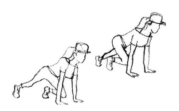

Mountain climbers.

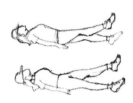

Flutter kicks.

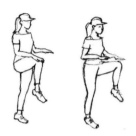

High knees running.

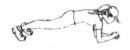

Plank.

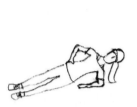

Side plank.

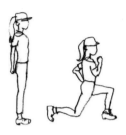

Lunges.

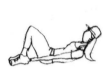

Heel touches.

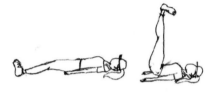

Leg raises.

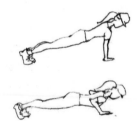

Push-ups.

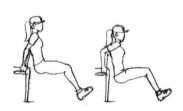

Tricep dips

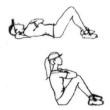

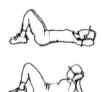

Sit-ups.   **Crunches.**

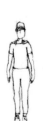
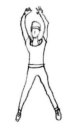

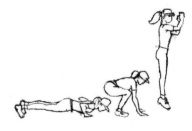

Jumping jacks.   **Burpees.**

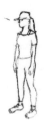

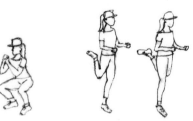

Squats.   **Butt kicks.**

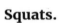

WANT MORE?

Now that you've **completed your 10-day challenge, guess what?** Here's some great news for you. You can move on to even shorter workouts. I know, right? If you've enjoyed these gym-free quick workouts and simple tasty meals, you'll love *Awesome at 50: Body Reboot in 6 weeks*. With more fuss-free, 5-19 minute long, 3-times-a-week exercises, the over-50s or *anyone* who wants to take back control of their health and fitness will find this book simple-to-follow, easy and helpful. Includes a delicious 30-day Asian-style meal plan with not much preparation required, saving you time and money. Read *Awesome at 50: Body Reboot in 6 weeks*.

Get organized with your routines. If you're trying to keep track of what you eat and how active you are so you can improve your diet and daily routines, then *Fitness and Meal Plan Journal: 12-Week Daily Workout and Food Planner Notebook* will be your friend and coach in your journey to becoming the healthier you. This no-nonsense, quick and easy-to-use organizer is available in a handy and portable 9" x 6" paperback format. Read *Fitness and Meal Plan Journal: 12-Week Daily Workout and Food Planner Notebook*.

BEFORE YOU GO

The book you are holding in your hand is the result of my dream to be an author. I hope you enjoyed it as much as I enjoyed writing it. I am slowly building my author brand, ranking and profile. As you probably suspected, it takes weeks, months or years to write a book. It exists through dedication, passion and love. Reviews help persuade others to give my books a shot. More readers will motivate me to write, which means more books. I love connecting with and hearing from you. I personally read each review you write. It gives me a sense of fulfilment and meaning— you read my book, I read your review. It will take *less than a minute* and can be just a line to say what you liked or didn't. If you could do me just this one favour and help me, I would be ever so grateful. Please leave me a review on Amazon USA or Amazon UK. A big thank you. *Ivy*

"The longer I live the more beautiful life becomes."
- Frank Lloyd Wright

ABOUT THE AUTHOR

I. Ngeow was born and raised in Johor Bahru, Malaysia. A graduate of the Middlesex University Writing MA programme, Ivy won the 2005 Middlesex University Literary Press Prize out of almost 1500 entrants worldwide. Her debut *Cry of the Flying Rhino* (2017) won the 2016 International Proverse Prize.

A regular suburban London mum who likes books, wine and cake, Ivy has had a passion for creative writing since she was a child, winning her first competition at 16. She started writing non-fiction lifestyle books to help families or busy and tired people, like herself, to save time and money by cooking and keeping fit at home in modern, quick and easy ways. Her interests include impromptu virtuoso piano performances, health and fitness, beauty and sewing. You can find her here:

writengeow (www.writengeow.com)
Twitter (twitter.com/ivyngeow)
Facebook (facebook.com/ivyngeowwriter)
Instagram (www.instagram.com/ivyngeow)
Email: ivy_ngeow AT yahoo DOT com

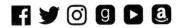

ALSO BY I. NGEOW

COOKBOOKS

30 Chinese Dinners: Healthy Easy Homemade Meals

Quick and Easy Party Treats: for special occasions

FITNESS

Fitness and Meal Plan Journal: 12-week daily workout and food planner notebook

Amazing at 50: 10-day Flat Tummy Challenge

Awesome at 50: Body Reboot in 6 weeks

DESIGN

Midcentury Modern: 15 Interior Design Ideas

ACKNOWLEDGMENTS

I WOULD LIKE TO thank my parents for giving me the genetics that I was born with. My family who taught me to love and to value life. I don't need a gym because they are my gym. My friends, my Instagram and Twitter followers who have become friends. You've always been there for me, supported my artistic endeavors and my pursuit of a life more meaningful. May we all live a beautiful life.

To all of you, my special thanks.

Printed in Great Britain
by Amazon